DK Natural Care Library
GINKGO
INCREASE INTELLECT & IMPROVE CIRCULATION

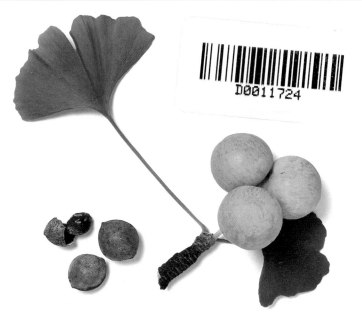

By STEPHANIE PEDERSEN

DORLING KINDERSLEY PUBLISHING, INC.
www.dk.com

CONTENTS

Conditions and Doses

HERBAL HISTORY

Long before over-the-counter medications and prescription drugs came on the scene, herbs proved to be powerful healers. Every culture on earth has used herbal medicine. In fact, herbal usage is older than recorded history itself: Herbal preparations were found in the burial site of a Neanderthal man who lived over 60,000 years ago.

When it comes to herbal medicine, many healing systems are available and useful. Perhaps the best known are ayurveda, Chinese medicine, and Western herbalism. Ayurveda is a system of diagnosis and treatment that uses herbs in conjunction with breathing, meditation, and yoga. It has been practiced in India for more than 2,500 years. Ayurveda gets its name from the Sanskrit words *ayuh*, meaning "longevity," and *veda*, meaning "knowledge." Indeed, in ayurvedic healing, health can be achieved only after identifying a person's physical and mental characteristics (called *dosha*). Then the proper preventative or therapeutic remedies are prescribed to help an individual maintain doshic balance.

Chinese medicine is another healing system that uses herbs, in combination with acupressure, acupuncture, and qi gong. Sometimes called traditional Chinese medicine (TCM), this ancient system is thought to be rooted as far back as 2,800 BC in the time of emperor Sheng Nung. Known as China's patron saint of herbal medicine, Sheng Nung is credited among the first proponents of healing plants. Chinese medicine attempts to help the body correct energy imbalances. Therefore herbs are classified according to certain active characteristics, such as heating, cooling, moisturizing, or drying, and prescribed according to how they influence the activity of various organ systems.

Many herbal practitioners believe that Western herbalism can trace its roots to the ancient Sumerians, who—according to a medicinal recipe dating from 3000 BC—boasted a refined knowledge of herbal medicine. Records from subsequent cultures, such as the Assyrians, Egyptians, Israelites, Greeks, and Romans, show similar herbal healing systems. But these peoples weren't the only ones using beneficial plants. The Celts, Gauls, Scandinavians, and other early European tribes also healed with herbs. In fact, it was their knowledge, melded with the medicine brought by invading Moors and Romans, that formed the foundation for Western herbalism. Simply put, this foundation formed a comprehensive system wherein herbs were grouped according to how they affected both the body and specific body systems.

Western herbalism was refined further when Europeans traveled to the New World. Once here, the Europeans fused their medical knowledge with that of the Native Americans. Herbal know-how became an important part of early American habits, so that wellness remedies were handed down from mothers to daughters to granddaughters, and medicinal plants were grown in home gardens. Physicians from the 1600s, 1700s, 1800s, and early 1900s commonly used plants, such as arnica, echinacea, and garlic to heal patients. Herbs were listed as medicine in official publications such as the *United States Pharmacopoeia* (the definitive American listing) and the *National Formulary* (the pharmacist's handbook). With the creation of synthetic medications in the 1930s, herbal medicine began to wane.

Fortunately, Europeans and Asians never gave up their herbal remedies. Instead, they used them to complement synthetic medications. Their successes—combined with the desire of many Americans for alternatives to the high price tags and unforgiving side effects of synthetic drugs—have kept the world moving forward on a healthier herbal path.

What Is Ginkgo?

Ginkgo has become a household word when it comes to herbs. Walk the aisles of any health store and you can't miss it: ginkgo in capsules, liquid extracts, tea, and more. Yet ginkgo is no medicinal newcomer—the herb boasts a long, distinguished history as an astringent, circulatory stimulant, expectorant and vasodilator. Centuries of Chinese healers have used it to fight such wide-ranging ills as asthma, bladder infections, chronic coughing, headaches, memory problems, premature ejaculation, and tuberculosis. In fact, some of the earliest recorded usages of the herb—to expel phlegm, strengthen the lungs, and relieve wheezing—come from emperors who lived and worked before Christ was born: Fu Si (2953–2838 BCE), Shen Nung (2838–2698 BCE) and Huang Di (2697–2595 BCE).

Commonly called ginkgo, ginkgo biloba grows in Australia, Europe and North America, but the tree is indigenous to China and neighboring countries. Extremely hardy, it thrives in a number of conditions, including urban parks and sidewalk planters, polluted air, drought, and areas of low sunlight. It is so hardy, in fact, that it lived right through the world's early Ice Age; as proof, archaeologists have found fossilized ginkgo trees from the Triassic portion of the Mesozoic era, some 200 million years ago. Furthermore, individual trees are capable of living nearly 4000 years, and there are currently many 1000- and 2000-year-old ginkgo trees in China, Japan and Korea.

A member of the Ginkgoaceae family,

ginkgo is a deciduous tree that can reach heights of 120 feet. It has leathery, fan-shaped leaves that turn gold in autumn, and smelly, apricot-sized fruits that house large seeds (sometimes called "kernels" or "nuts"). In North America and Europe, it is the tree's leaves that are employed medicinally. Although the leaves are also utilized in Asia, the seeds and seed oil are more commonly used.

Today, ginkgo is best known as a brain function booster that is especially helpful in combating "cerebral vascular insufficiency illnesses" which are so common among the elderly of developed nations. These types of mental illnesses are caused by atherosclerosis of the cerebral arteries (thanks to rich diets heavy with animal fats) and include dementia, greatly impaired thinking, senility, short-term memory loss and slowed mental response. Among the herb's compounds are flavone glycosides and terpene lactones, which work together to dilate blood vessels, increase blood circulation and inhibit coagulation. Together, these three actions encourage blood flow to the brain. How does all this aid mental function? Simple: When blood flow to the brain is weakened, the brain's tissues receive less nourishing oxygen, which in turn impairs normal functioning. Increase oxygen-rich blood to brain tissues, and the brain functions better.

Yet mental conditions aren't all ginkgo is good for. The herb helps prevent or treat other illnesses produced by diminished blood flow, including impotence, gangrene as a symptom of diabetes, leg cramping and thrombosis. Furthermore, the above-mentioned flavone glycosides and terpene lactones, plus the ingredient quercetin (which is an extremely potent free radical scavenger), boast strong antioxidant, free radical-scavenging and membrane-stabilizing effects to help protect blood vessels, brain, eyes, and heart against destructive free radicals.

IN OTHER WORDS
Like many herbs, Ginkgo is known by several names. Here are a few of them:

❊ **Bai Guo**
❊ **Ginkgo Biloba**
❊ **Kew Tree**
❊ **Maidenhair Tree**
❊ **Silver Apricot**
❊ **Yin Guo**
❊ **Ying Xing**

SCIENCE TALK

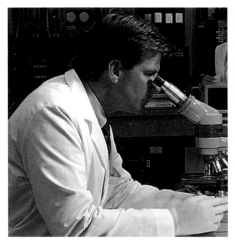

MEDICINE WORLDWIDE
The National Institutes of Health, in Bethesda, MD, estimate that only 10 to 30 percent of the health care worldwide is allopathic, or "Western." The rest of the world's medical care is what Americans would call "alternative," including ayurveda, energy healing, herbalism, homeopathy and traditional Chinese medicine.

CELEBRATING GERMAN KNOW-HOW
Perhaps no other country in the Western world has done more than Germany to further the cause of herbal medicine. What's the country's secret? Commission E, a review board of respected pharmacologists, physicians and scientists. The board was established in 1978, and members spent the first 15 years researching more than 300 age-old herbal remedies for usages, recommended dosages, preparations and side effects. Then, in 1980, the German government upped the medical ante, creating a mandate requiring all new herbal remedies sold in pharmacies to meet the same criteria as over-the-counter drugs. To comply, researchers performed thousands of rigorous clinical trials, resulting in a deep well of knowledge used by doctors open to herbs worldwide.

DO YOU HAVE A CONTRAINDICATION?

Before taking any herb, it's important to ask your physician whether you have any contraindications.

What does contraindication mean? It's a common medical term that refers to a symptom or condition that makes a particular treatment inadvisable. For example, when it comes to ginko, hemophilia is a contraindication. Why? Adding the vasodilating powers of ginko to this mix can create an even greater health hazard.

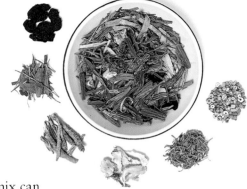

Before taking any herb, ask yourself the following questions:

✔ Have I done any background research on the herb?

✔ What condition am I taking this herb for?

✔ Am I taking other medications or herbs that may affect the herb's functioning?

✔ Do I have any preexisting condition that is contraindicated?

✔ Am I pregnant, trying to conceive or nursing?

✔ Have I spoken to my physician, a naturopathic doctor or an herbalist before taking herb?

✔ Do I know the proper dosages for the herb?

RETHINKING MEDICATION

ANTIBIOTICS: ARE THEY ESSENTIAL?

A recent report published in the *Journal of the American Medical Association* stated that even though antibiotics provide little help for colds, upper respiratory tract infections and bronchitis, doctors still prescribe antibiotics for these conditions. Why? In part, because patients expect their doctors to give them some kind of medication, and many physicians find it easier to oblige than take time out to explain how antibiotics do and don't work. Americans are so enamored of antibiotics that doctors write over 12 million antibiotic prescriptions annually. To learn more about the dangers of antibiotic abuse, contact the Centers For Disease Control and Prevention, 404-332-4555.

PENICILLIN BY THE POUND

Since penicillin's debut in 1941, antibiotic production has shot up from 2 million pounds in 1954 to more than 50 million pounds in 1997. Where is all this medication going? Half of the antibiotics produced annually are prescribed for people; the rest are mixed into livestock feed and used as fertilizers for agricultural crops. The downside to this free-flowing penicillin? New, strong, antibiotic-resistant strains of bacteria.

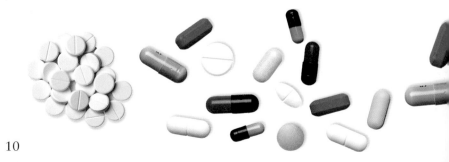

WAIT! BEFORE YOU TAKE THAT PILL . . .

Before asking your doctor for an antibiotic, ask yourself the following questions:

✔ Is my condition caused by bacteria? If not, antibiotics will not work.

✔ Are antibiotics necessary for recovery? If the infection will go away on its own, consider forgoing antibiotics.

✔ Are there alternatives to antibiotics? If herbal or other natural remedies can fight off the infection, consider using one or more of them.

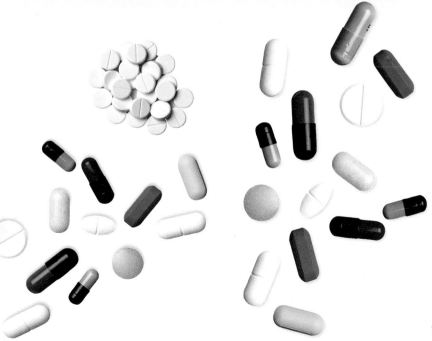

COMMON SIDE EFFECTS

Like many medicinal herbs, ginkgo can cause mild side effects. Here's what a small number of users experience:

✔ **Dizziness.** Though it is an extremely rare side effect, a very small number of individuals experience minor dizziness when taking ginkgo.

✔ **Gastrointestinal Upsets.** Ginkgo has been shown to cause minor stomach upset in up to 4 percent of individuals.

✔ **Headache.** Though it is an extremely rare side effect, a very small number of individuals experience mild headaches when taking ginkgo.

WHAT TO LOOK FOR?
In the market for a ginkgo remedy, but you're not sure how to choose one? The most effective remedies boast a high concentration of the active ingredients flavone glycosides and terpene lactones. To ensure you get the most potent—and beneficial—medicine available, look for products standardized to 24 percent flavone glycoside and 6 percent terpene per dose.

PRECAUTIONS

✖ The doses in this book are generally aimed at adults. We strongly suggest consulting your child's physician before administering ginkgo externally or internally. If your physician does okay ginkgo for your child, we generally recommend halving the adult doses suggested in this book. Again, please consult your child's physician.

✖ Do not self-medicate with ginkgo while taking any type of anticoagulant medication. To do so can thin the blood too much, leading to possible internal bleeding. For information on how to safely switch from a synthetic anticoagulant to ginkgo, talk to your physician.

✖ Do not self-medicate with ginkgo while taking any type of vasodilator medication. To do so can overdilate blood vessels. For information on how to safely switch from a synthetic anticoagulant to ginkgo, talk to your physician.

✖ If you are pregnant, nursing, trying to conceive or are taking any type of medication, please consult your physician before using ginkgo.

✖ To avoid dangerous interactions between prescription medication and herbal medicine, individuals with AIDS, cancer, a connective tissue disease, heart disease, kidney disease, liver disease, tuberculosis, or any other chronic illness should consult their physician before using any herb.

FORMULA GUIDE

Capsules, extracts, teas, tinctures—what do they all mean?
For the uninitiated, we offer this guide to herbal formulas:

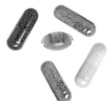

❊ **Capsules.** The medicinal part of the herb is freeze-dried, pulverized and packed into gelatin capsules. Ginkgo capsules usually contain 40 mg to 120 mg of herb powder; occasionally the dried herb is reinforced with concentrated extracts.

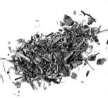

❊ **Herb, Dried.** The flowers, leaves, stems and/or roots of many herbs are often available dried at health food stores and herbal pharmacies. While these are most commonly made into homemade teas, they can also be used to make decoctions, infused oils, sachets and more.

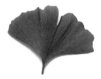

❊ **Herb, Fresh.** Herbs that are used in both culinary and medicinal ways (such as parsley or dill) are most often found fresh. These can be made into homemade extract, juice, infused oil, tea and more.

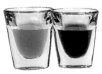

❊ **Juices.** The extracted juice from fresh herbs can be found mixed with commercially prepared fruit or vegetable juices.

❊ **Liquid Extract** (also called Extract). Macerated plant material is steeped over a period of time in a solvent or solvents such as alcohol, glycerin and/or water. The steeped liquid is then reduced to lessen the concentration of (or entirely remove) the solvents. Generally stronger than a tincture.

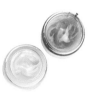

❖ **Oil, Essential** (also called Oil). Essential oils are the volatile oily components of herbs. They are found in tiny glands located in the flowers, leaves, roots and/or bark and are mechanically or chemically extracted. Essential oil is prescribed almost exclusively for external use.

❖ **Oil, Infused.** Made by steeping fresh or dried herbs in an edible oil. After a period of time, the herbs are removed and the oil used internally or externally. Not as potent as essential oil.

❖ **Ointments.** Dried or fresh herbs are steeped in a base of oils and emulsifiers (such as beeswax, petroleum jelly or soft paraffin wax). After a period of time, the herbs are removed and the ointment packaged. For external use only.

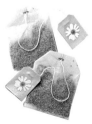

❖ **Syrups.** Syrups are generally a combination of herbal extracts and a sweetener, such as honey or sugar. Generally used for colds, flu and sore throats.

❖ **Teas/Infusions.** The words "tea" and "infusion" are often used interchangeably in herbal healing. While commercial herbal tea bags are available, herbal tea can also be made with loose dried or fresh herbs.

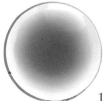

❖ **Tinctures.** Plant material is soaked in alcohol. The saturated plant material is then pressed. Liquid from this pressing may be diluted with water and packaged—usually in small dropper bottles.

CONDITIONS AND DOSES

ASTHMA

❏ **Symptoms:** Asthma is an inflammation of the airways. It is caused by an allergic reaction and affects almost 10 million Americans. Although not all sufferers are allergic to the same substances, some common triggers are animal dander, dust mites, mold spores and pollen. When a trigger is inhaled, the body's antibodies react with the allergen, producing allergen-suppressing histamine and other chemicals. Also, chest muscles constrict, the bronchial lining becomes inflamed and the body creates more mucous, thus causing breathing difficulties, coughing (sometimes accompanied by mucus), painless tightness in the chest and wheezing.

❏ **How Ginkgo Can Help:** The ginkgolides in ginkgo have been shown in clinical studies to inhibit the chemical mediator that produces asthma attacks. Meanwhile, the herb's much-touted anti-inflammatory ability helps shrink swollen bronchial lining so asthmatics can breathe.

❏ **Dosages:** For individuals who suffer from frequent asthma attacks, ginkgo can be a preventative when taken as one 40-mg capsule, three times a day with meals; or 1/2 teaspoon of liquid extract, three times a day before meals; or 1 teaspoon of tincture, three times a day before meals. For individuals whose asthma attacks occur less frequently, 600 mg of ginkgo can be taken immediately at the first sign of symptoms.

RESPIRATORY ALLERGIES

❏ **Symptoms:** A respiratory allergy feels similar to a cold—only with more itchiness. The condition is an immune-system response to a specific airborne allergen, usually animal dander, dust, mold or pollen. When the allergen is inhaled, an allergic person produces antibodies, which react with the offending substance and prompt the release of histamine. Histamine causes the lining of the nose, sinuses, eyelids and eyes to become inflamed, causing a variety of symptoms, including coughing, frequent sneezing, itchiness at the roof of the mouth, itchy eyes, itchy nose, itchy throat, runny nose, stuffy nose and watery eyes. Interestingly, when a person is allergic to pollen, the allergy is sometimes called hay fever—even though allergies to airborne dander, dust and mold produce identical symptoms.

❏ **How Ginkgo Can Help:** The ginkgolides in ginkgo have been shown in clinical studies to inhibit the chemical mediator that produces allergic reactions. Meanwhile, the herb's much-touted anti-inflammatory ability helps shrink swollen nasal and sinus linings so the allergy sufferer can breathe.

❏ **Dosages:** For individuals who are in frequent contact with their "trigger allergen," ginkgo can be a preventative when taken as one 40-mg capsule, three times a day with meals; or 1/2 teaspoon of liquid extract, three times a day before meals; or 1 teaspoon of tincture, three times a day before meals. For individuals whose contact with their allergen is less frequent, 600 mg of ginkgo can be taken an hour before anticipated contact, or immediately upon contact.

CONDITIONS AND DOSES

CLAUDIFICATION (LEG CRAMPS)

❏ **Symptoms:** When blood doesn't flow freely to the lower legs, painful cramps can develop, making it difficult to walk or stand. Called claudification after the limping Roman emperor Claudius, the condition occurs when the arteries leading to the leg become blocked with fatty deposits, or when the arteries' linings become inflamed. A diet heavy in animal fats is responsible in the first instance, while inactivity or smoking are generally to blame in the second.

❏ **How Ginkgo Can Help:** In France and Germany, ginkgo is routinely prescribed for claudification. A French study found that in 75 percent of claudification patients, the herb increased blood flow to the lower leg. Just how does ginkgo do this? Two of its constituents, flavone glycosides and terpene lactones, dilate inflamed or blocked arteries so blood can reach the lower legs. In cases where claudification is caused by inflammation, these substances can also reduce swelling. Furthermore, the flavonoids that are in ginkgo help tissue regenerate by killing free radicals that were created by lack of oxygen to the affected areas.

❏ **Dosages:** Take one 40-mg capsule three times a day with meals; or 1/2 teaspoon of liquid extract, three times a day before meals; or 1 teaspoon of tincture, three times a day before meals. Expect to begin seeing results after four weeks. Ginkgo can be taken indefinitely.

CORONARY ARTERY DISEASE

❒ **Symptoms:** Coronary artery disease accounts for about 1 in 2 American deaths each year. The disease progresses slowly over the course of years and even decades, but its impact can be instantaneous: In nearly a third of all cases, death occurs without any previous warning of disease. Indeed, some people have no symptoms, while others may experience chest pain, constriction or a sense of heaviness in the chest, fatigue, pallor, shortness of breath, swelling in the ankles and/or weakness. Coronary artery disease occurs when cholesterol deposits build up on coronary artery walls. These special blood vessels provide oxygen and nutrients to the muscles of the heart. When they are unable to deliver adequate blood flow, the heart muscle begins to weaken, leading to angina (chest pain), congestive heart failure, and heart attack. When it comes to causes, a high-fat diet is most often implicated, although heredity, stress, inactivity, smoking and alcoholism are also culprits.

❒ **How Ginkgo Can Help:** Several studies have shown that ginkgo combats coronary artery disease in a number of ways. The antioxidant flavonoids help kill the artery-damaging free radicals created by cholesterol deposits. Flavone glycosides and terpene lactones dilate blocked arteries so blood can reach the heart. These two elements also keep blood platelets from becoming sticky and thick; thin blood can more easily pass through blocked arteries.

❒ **Dosages:** If you are currently being treated for coronary artery disease, do not take ginkgo without first consulting your cardiologist. If given the go-ahead, take one 40-mg capsule, three times a day with meals; or 1/2 teaspoon of liquid extract, three times a day before meals; or 1 teaspoon of tincture, three times a day.

CONDITIONS AND DOSES

HYPERTENSION

❒ **Symptoms:** Hypertension, more commonly known as high blood pressure, is a condition in which blood travels through the arteries at higher pressure than normal. This increased blood flow literally wears out the blood vessels, heart and kidneys and can lead to premature death. What causes hypertension? Cigarettes, alcohol, some medications and certain illnesses can elevate blood pressure— but by far the most common cause of hypertension is clogged arteries from a high-fat diet. When blood vessels are blocked with fatty deposits, the heart must work harder to move the same amount of blood through them. This in turn increases the pressure at which the blood is pumped. Unfortunately, hypertension is symptomless, leaving many individuals unaware that they even suffer from the condition—until it's too late.

❒ **How Ginkgo Can Help:** Flavone glycosides and terpene lactones work in two ways to treat hypertension: They dilate blood vessels so blood can more easily pass through, and they inhibit coagulation so blood doesn't clog on deposits as it moves through the veins.

❒ **Dosages:** Take one 40-mg capsule, three times a day with meals; or 1/2 teaspoon of liquid extract, three times a day before meals; or 1 teaspoon of tincture, three times a day before meals. Expect to begin seeing results after four weeks. Ginkgo can be taken indefinitely.

GINKGO AND CHINESE MEDICINE

In Traditional Chinese Medicine, ginkgo is used to treat illnesses caused by damp heat, deficient kidney yin, or deficient lung qi. Just what kind of illnesses would these be? Here's a rundown:

❊ **Damp Heat** imbalances often appear as skin conditions. Abscesses, boils, chicken pox, herpes, infected sores, lesions and shingles are examples. Internal damp heat conditions involve the upper respiratory tract.

❊ **Deficient Kidney Yin** can cause dry mouth and throat, excessive thirst, flushed skin, hot hands and feet, insomnia, lower-back pain, night sweats, ringing in the ears or premature ejaculation.

❊ **Deficient Lung Qi** is characterized by the following: allergies, asthma, chilliness, general weakness, shallow cough, shallow respiration, sparse white phlegm, susceptibility to colds, sweating, weak or soft voice.

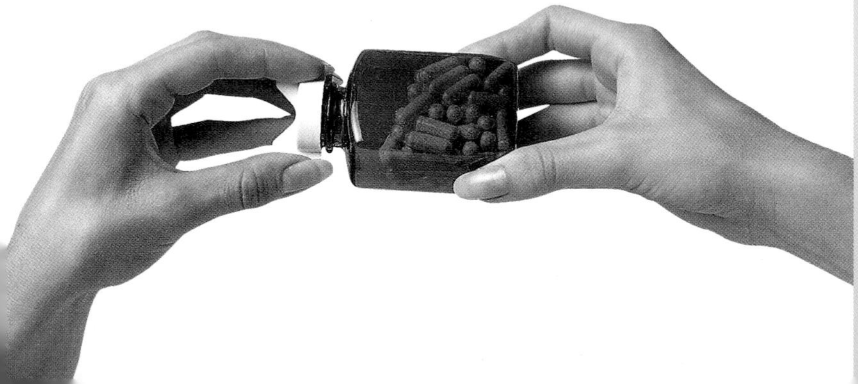

CONDITIONS AND DOSES

TINNITUS

❏ **Symptoms:** Individuals with tinnitus hear some type of noise in one ear—usually buzzing, hissing, ringing, roaring or whistling—when no such noise is present in the environment around them. These noises may be continuous or intermittent, they may or may not be synchronized with the heartbeat, they may range from soft to loud and they may be accompanied by hearing loss. Tinnitus is usually a secondary symptom of a variety of conditions, including acoustic trauma, Ménière's disease, middle ear infection, occupational hearing loss, or wax buildup. Sometimes, however, tinnitus occurs spontaneously with no explanation.

❏ **How Ginkgo Can Help:** Ginkgo has been shown in French studies to lessen or eradicate tinnitus. It is believed that the herb works in three ways: improving blood circulation to the ear; strengthening nerve connections between the ear and brain; and fighting off age-related free radicals that can damage nerve cells in the ear.

❏ **Dosages:** Take one 40-mg capsule, three times a day with meals; or 1/2 teaspoon of liquid extract, three times a day before meals; or 1 teaspoon of tincture, three times a day before meals. Expect to see mild results within two weeks, stronger results in six to eight weeks. Ginkgo can be taken indefinitely.

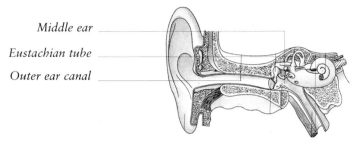

Middle ear

Eustachian tube

Outer ear canal

Tinnitus is usually a secondary symptom of a variety of conditions, including acoustic trauma, Ménière's disease, middle ear infection, occupational hearing loss or wax buildup.

GINKGO AROUND THE WORLD

To the Germans and French, ginkgo is a highly regarded treatment for Alzheimer's disease, depression, circulatory disorders, hearing problems and memory loss so highly regarded, in fact, that 1.5 million prescriptions for the herb are written every week. In Germany, the herb accounts for 1 percent of all prescription medication and in France it accounts for 4 percent. In fact, in one year the two countries' combined sales of ginkgo were more than $500 million.

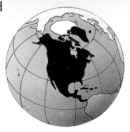

CONDITIONS AND DOSES

AGE-RELATED MACULAR DEGENERATION

❏ **Symptoms:** Also known as involutional macular degeneration or senile degeneration, this is the most frequent cause of legal blindness in the United States and Great Britain. The macula, which is the central portion of the retina, is responsible for central vision. As some people age, however, the layer of insulation between the retina and the blood vessels behind it begins to break down, making it easy for fluid to leak into the retina from the blood vessels. As a result of this damage, scar tissue begins to form on the macula, creating a corresponding blind spot. This scar tissue begins to spread, thus creating an increasingly larger blind area in an individual's field of vision. While a person's peripheral vision is largely unaffected, it becomes more difficult for the individual to see what lies straight ahead. Experts believe that damage done by free radicals is what causes age-related macular degeneration.

❏ **How Ginkgo Can Help:** Ginkgo is regularly used in France and Germany as a treatment for macular degeneration. A French study of patients with macular degeneration proved ginkgo successful in improving central vision. How? Ginkgo's flavonoids help reverse free radical damage, which is believed to cause macular degeneration.

❏ **Dosages:** Studies have shown that once 20 percent or more of a person's vision is lost to macular degeneration, that vision cannot be returned. For this reason, consider taking ginkgo has a preventative: one 40-mg capsule, three times a day with meals; or 1/2 teaspoon of liquid extract three times a day before meals; or 1 teaspoon of tincture three times a day before meals. If you already have signs of macular degeneration, you can diminish or prevent further damage by taking two 40-mg capsules three times a day with meals; or 1 teaspoon of liquid extract three times a day before meals; or 2 teaspoons of tincture three times a day before meals. Ginkgo can be taken indefinitely.

GINKGO: ANTI-AGING MEDICATION?
In medical circles, one of the most famous studies on ginkgo was conducted in France and published in the September 1986 issue of *La Presse Médicale*. French researchers examined 166 geriatric patients for 17 markers: ability to walk, appetite, anxiety, cooperation, depression, disturbances in orientation, emotional stability, fatigue, headache, initiative, personal care, ringing in the ears, short-term memory, sleep abnormalities, sociability, vertigo and vivacity. After taking 160 mg of ginkgo every day for three months, all test subjects— regardless of their beginning state— made mild to excellent improvement in all 17 areas.

CONDITIONS AND DOSES

HEMORRHOIDS

❐ **Symptoms:** A membrane lines the lowest part of the anus and rectum. Just under this membrane are clusters of veins. Sometimes, these veins become swollen—perhaps as a result of pregnancy, chronic constipation or straining during a bowel movement. Regardless of the cause, these swollen veins are called hemorrhoids. Symptoms of the condition can include anal itching, tenderness (especially during a bowel movement), protrusion of soft tissue at the anus and bright red blood on toilet paper or stool after a bowel movement.

❐ **How Ginkgo Can Help:** A French study found that ginkgo was effective in lessening symptoms of acute and chronic hemorrhoids in 86 percent of patients. Ginkgo has powerful anti-inflammatory abilities that can reduce the swelling that causes hemorrhoids.

❐ **Dosages:** Apply ginkgo poultice or fomentation directly to affected area up to three times a day, or swab the area up to three times a day with ginkgo tea. Taken internally, ginkgo also helps shrink hemorrhoids. Take one 40-mg capsule three times a day with meals; or 1/2 to 1 teaspoon of liquid extract three times a day before meals; or 1 to 2 teaspoons of tincture three times a day before meals. Discontinue when hemorrhoid has healed.

USING MORE THAN THE LEAVES

In using this book, you'll notice we focus on ginkgo leaf formulas. That's because Western research and usage has concentrated solely on this part of the tree. Yet, the leaves aren't the only medicinal portion of the plant. In China, Korea and Japan, doctors use ginkgo seeds for complaints linked to "wind-damp" illnesses. These ailments include allergies, asthma, bladder infections, blisters, boils, chills, colds, fever, heaviness in the chest, heaviness in the head, influenza, joint pain, muscle cramps, skin rashes, sparse urination, tuberculosis and uterine cramps. The seeds, which are mildly toxic in their raw state, are boiled and dried. They can be ground and taken as a powder or swallowed in capsule form, but more often they are left whole and eaten alone or added to food. In late autumn it is common to see Chinese men and women in New York's Central Park, scooping up the ginkgo fruit that has fallen to the ground from the city's trees. Because the plum-like fruit encapsulating the seeds can cause a poison-ivy-like rash, gloves are worn while harvesting. Canned ginkgo seeds can be bought in most Chinese neighborhoods, where the kernels are added to recipes. For more information on using ginkgo seeds, please contact a qualified doctor of Chinese medicine.

CONDITIONS AND DOSES

IMPOTENCE

❏ **Symptoms:** While anything from too much alcohol to anger to depression can cause short-term erectile problems, impotence is defined as a chronic inability to have or sustain an erection. It is believed that as many as 30 million American men suffer from the condition. In 90 percent of the cases, an organic cause is the culprit—usually diminished blood flow caused by fatty deposits in the arteries leading from the heart to the penis.

❏ **How Ginkgo Can Help:** In Chinese medicine, ginkgo is regularly prescribed to treat impotence. Indeed, several American studies of impotent men have found ginkgo effective in restoring blood flow to the penis, thereby helping patients to achieve and maintain erections. The herb does this by dilating blood vessels, thus allowing blood to more easily reach the penis. In rare cases, impotence is caused by low levels of testosterone, produced in the testes. Overall glandular functions are controlled by the pituitary.

❏ **Dosages:** Take one 40-mg capsule three times a day with meals; or 1/2 to 1 teaspoon of liquid extract three times a day before meals; or 1 to 2 teaspoons of tincture three times a day before meals. Expect to see results in six to eight weeks. Ginkgo can be taken infinitely.

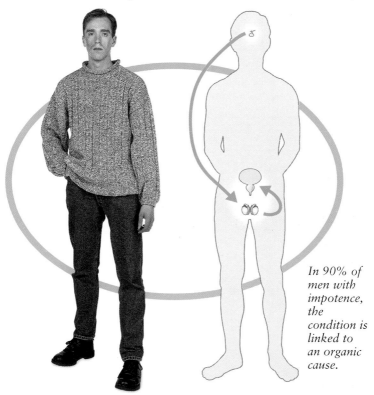

In 90% of men with impotence, the condition is linked to an organic cause.

CONDITIONS AND DOSES

ALZHEIMER'S DISEASE

❏ **Symptoms:** How many times have you heard someone mistakenly call Alzheimer's disease "old-timer's disease"? The mistake is a natural one, considering that Alzheimer's primarily strikes older adults. While the disease can strike people in their 40s or 50s, it most commonly affects those aged 65 and older. In fact, about every 1 in 10 people over the age of 65 is diagnosed with Alzheimer's, and studies show that over four million Americans have the disease. Alzheimer's is an incurable disease that destroys brain cells—usually those of the cerebral cortex—causing dementia. Symptoms appear progressively, usually in this order: forgetfulness, shortened attention span, disintegration of personality, disorientation, memory loss, confusion, restlessness, inability to read, wandering, lack of patience, loss of impulse control, inappropriate behavior, aggressiveness, irritability, cursing, lack of coordination, delusions, hallucinations, loss of language, lack of bladder and bowel control, and inability to feed oneself. Currently, there is no diagnostic test for Alzheimer's; the most foolproof test for the disease is an autopsy to examine brain tissue. That said, physicians can make an accurate diagnosis in up to 90 percent of all cases after a careful medical history and physical examination. It's not known exactly what causes Alzheimer's. Some researches believe it is an inflammatory response to infection; others blame it on free radicals, environmental toxins, or lack of blood flow to the brain. Whatever the culprit, genetics is often a factor.

❏ **How Ginkgo Can Help:** Right now there is no cure for Alzheimer's disease, although several studies have shown that ginkgo can delay the onset of the disease or lessen its severity. In a recent German study, 216 patients with mild to moderate Alzheimer's disease were divided into two groups. One group received 240 mg of ginkgo a day the other group received a placebo. At the end of one month, the group taking ginkgo showed increased mental alertness and decreased irritability while the placebo group remained the same. Other studies have shown that Alzheimer's patients taking ginkgo for four to eight weeks have an increase in the turnover of norepinephrine (an important chemical transmitter) in the brain, indicating increased brain activity.

❒ **Dosages:** Two 40-mg capsules three times a day with meals; or 1/2 to 1 teaspoon of liquid extract three times a day before meals; or 1 to 2 teaspoons of tincture three times a day before meals. Expect to begin seeing results after four weeks. Ginkgo can be taken indefinitely.

DEMENTIA VS. ALZHEIMER'S DISEASE— WHAT'S THE DIFFERENCE?

The word "dementia" refers to a gradual loss of mental functioning, regardless of its cause. Dementia is not a disease but a syndrome, meaning it is characterized by a group of symptoms that can include a gradual loss of short-term memory, inability to learn new information, growing tendency to repeat oneself, misplacing objects, confusion, getting lost, slow disintegration of personality, loss of judgment, lack of social graces, increasing irritability, restlessness and lack of bowel and/or bladder function. Alzheimer's, on the other hand, is an actual disease—a disease that causes dementia. Other conditions that can produce dementia are Huntington's disease, multiple sclerosis, Parkinson's disease, AIDS, stroke, and brain damage caused by trauma.

CONDITIONS AND DOSES

DYSTHYMIA

❏ **Symptoms:** Dysthymia, from the Greek *dysthymia*, translates as "bad mood." In medical-speak, however, the term refers to mild to moderate depression. The condition often begins with no apparent trigger, though it can also develop from a specific incident. Symptoms can include change in appetite, decreased self-esteem, grief, helplessness, impaired daily functioning, irritability, loss of interest in once-enjoyable activities, inappropriate guilt, lethargy, neglect of physical appearance, malaise, self-reproach, sense of doom, sleep disturbances, slowed physical and mental responses, social withdrawal and thoughts of suicide.

❏ **How Ginkgo Can Help:** The German Ministry of Health Committee for Herbal Remedies approves ginkgo for improving mood and mental processes, and several German studies have found ginkgo to be an effective antidepressant. In fact, one study found that individuals (aged 51 to 78) who did not respond to pharmaceutical antidepressants showed marked improvement after four weeks when given 240 mg of ginkgo daily. The herb helps combat depression in two ways: by increasing blood flow to the brain for more efficient brain functioning, and by increasing brain levels of dopamine. A neurotransmitter, dopamine helps regulate mood and is critical to the transfer of information among nerves.

❐ **Dosages:** When taken on a daily basis, two 40-mg capsules, three times a day with meals; or 1/2 to 1 teaspoon of liquid extract three times a day before meals; or 1 to 2 teaspoons of tincture, 3 times a day before meals. Expect to see mild results within two weeks, stronger results in four to eight weeks.

RADIATION

Ginkgo contains a group of ingredients known as flavonoids, the major ones of which are quercetin, kaempferol and isorhamnetine. These substances are intense antioxidants, able to fight off the most aggressive onslaught of free radicals. That's why the herb is sometimes used by scientists to counteract the effects of radiation. One of the most celebrated examples of this came after the 1987 malfunction of the Chernobyl nuclear power plant in what was then the Soviet Union. Researchers studied 30 workers responsible for dismantling the plant and cleaning up the toxic waste. Exposure to nuclear radiation had left each individual with greatly damaged chromosomes, which in turn put the group at high risk for cancer. In an effort to administer a treatment free of side effects, physicians decided upon ginkgo. Each worker received 40 mg of ginkgo, 3 times a day. At the end of two months, all were found to have greatly normalized chromosomes.

CONDITIONS AND DOSES

IMPAIRED CONCENTRATION

❏ **Symptoms:** Weakened concentration is often associated with aging—and with good reason. Individuals who have spent a lifetime eating a diet heavy in animal products often have cerebral arteries that are hardened and coated with plaque. The result: Less oxygen-rich blood is able to reach the brain. Without this nourishment, a number of the brain's mental functions can become impaired, concentration included. However, clogged blood vessels aren't the only concentration-stealer. Younger individuals who are besieged with stress, who are inactive, sleep-deficient, or drink heavily—all of which can temporarily slow blood flow to the brain—can also suffer from reduced concentration. Regardless of the cause, impaired concentration is characterized by an inability or reduced ability to concentrate during conversations and lectures and difficulty focusing on work tasks and written material.

❏ **How Ginkgo Can Help:** Flavone glycosides and terpene lactones work together to dilate blood vessels, increase blood circulation and inhibit blood coagulation. Together, these three actions encourage blood flow to the brain for improved mental functioning.

❏ **Dosages:** Take one 40-mg capsule, three times a day with meals; or 1/2 teaspoon of liquid extract three times a day before meals; or 1 teaspoon of tincture three times a day before meals. Expect to see mild results within two weeks, stronger results in six to eight weeks. Ginkgo can be taken indefinitely.

The ability to concentrate decreases when individuals of any age, including young people, have more stress than they can handle, drink heavily perhaps in an attempt to make themselves feel better, and don't get enough physical exercise or sleep.

CONDITIONS AND DOSES

IMPAIRED SHORT-TERM MEMORY

❏ **Symptoms:** Memory is a complex process that we still don't completely understand. How is it that you can remember your first day of kindergarten but can't for the life of you remember where you left your sunglasses this morning? And why is it that as we age, we often become even more forgetful of those things that just occurred? Scientists aren't sure exactly what's behind these temporary glitches in our memory banks. They know, however, that many older individuals have experienced a lifetime of fat-heavy meals, resulting in hardened, plaque-coated cerebral arteries. When this occurs, less oxygen-rich blood is able to reach the brain. Without this nourishment, a number of the brain's mental functions can become impaired, memory included. However, clogged blood vessels aren't the only memory stealer. Younger individuals who are besieged with stress, who are inactive, sleep-deficient, or drink heavily—all of which can temporarily slow blood flow to the brain—can also suffer from impaired short-term memory.

❏ **How Ginkgo Can Help:** Bulgarian, English, French, and German researchers have all conducted separate studies that show ginkgo to be helpful in combating reduced short-term memory. The constituents flavone glycosides and terpene lactones work together to dilate blood vessels, increase blood circulation and inhibit blood coagulation. Together, these three actions encourage blood flow to the brain for improved mental functioning.

❐ **Dosages:** When taken on a daily basis, one or two 40-mg capsules three times a day with meals; or 1/2 to 1 teaspoon of liquid extract three times a day before meals; or 1 to 2 teaspoons of tincture three times a day before meals. Expect to see mild results within two weeks, stronger results in six to 12 weeks. Ginkgo can be taken indefinitely.

TEST-TAKING SMARTS

You spend hours studying for an important exam, only to forget every drop of information come test time. Sound familiar? Next time you've got an examination to cram for, a speech to memorize, or lines to learn for your starring role in a community play, look to ginkgo for help. In French studies of short-term usage, the herb was found safe, effective and without side effects when taken at a high dosage (600 mg) one hour before studying. Although lower dosages (120 mg and 240 mg) are routinely prescribed for permanent memory impairment, they were shown to be ineffective when used as a temporary study aid. That said, daily high dosages of ginkgo should not be taken for long periods of time. While studies have yet to uncover hazards, there is the remote possibility that long-term, elevated daily doses of ginkgo can thin the blood to unhealthy levels. Better to limit 600-mg doses to the occasional weekly study session. To further maximize your ability to absorb information, don't study when tired or hungry, and avoid studying in noisy environments. Experts say you can also boost your brainpower by breaking up study periods into increments: Spend 20 to 40 minutes examining material before stopping for a 10-minute stretch. When you return to your books, spend 10 minutes reviewing what you've learned. Repeat as needed with additional material.

CONDITIONS AND DOSES

MIGRAINE HEADACHES

❏ **Symptoms:** Also called vascular headaches, migraines are extremely painful headaches that occur when cerebral blood vessels constrict, allowing less blood to reach the brain. The one constant symptom is severe head pain—often so extreme that individuals become nauseated and vomit. The pain typically begins on one side of the head and may gradually spread and throb. Migraines are usually preceded by several warning signs. Two to eight hours before the migraine occurs, some people may experience elation, drowsiness, intense thirst, irritability and a craving for sweets. About 15 to 30 minutes before the migraine occurs, some people may see an "aura," a group of symptoms that can include blank spots within the field of vision, dizziness, sparkling flashes of light, temporary numbness or paralysis of one side of the body and zigzag lines that cross the field of vision. It is not known why some people get migraines, although stress, alcohol consumption, specific foods and oral contraceptives can trigger cerebral vessels to constrict in some individuals, causing vascular headaches.

❏ **How Ginkgo Can Help:** Ginkgo is a vasodilator. In other words, it dilates constricted blood vessels so blood can flow smoothly. Several studies have shown that ginkgo's vasodilating action helps to relieve migraines.

❏ **Dosages:** For individuals who suffer from frequent migraines, ginkgo can be a preventative when taken as one 40-mg capsule three times a day with meals; or 1/2 teaspoon of liquid extract three times a day before meals; or 1 teaspoon of tincture three times a day before meals.

For individuals whose migraines occur less frequently, 600 mg of ginkgo can be taken immediately at the first sign of migraine symptoms.

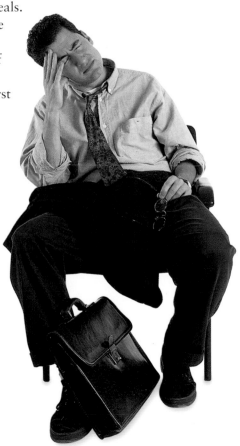

CONDITIONS AND DOSES

PREMENSTRUAL SYNDROME

❏ **Symptoms:** Premenstrual syndrome, popularly known as PMS, is a predictable pattern of physical and emotional changes that occur in some women just before menstruation. Symptoms range from barely noticeable to extreme and can include abdominal swelling, anxiety, bloating, breast soreness, clumsiness, depressed mood, difficulty concentrating, fatigue, fluid retention, headaches, irritability, lethargy, skin eruptions, sleep disturbances, swollen hands and feet and weight gain.

❏ **How Ginkgo Can Help:** Several American and French studies have shown ginkgo's anti-inflammatory powers to help in reducing the swelling, breast soreness and fluid retention associated with PMS. Furthermore, the herb combats headaches by boosting blood circulation to the brain.

❏ **Dosages:** Two weeks before your period, begin taking one 40-mg capsule three times a day with meals; or 1/4 teaspoon liquid extract three times a day with meals; or 1/2 teaspoon tincture three times a day with meals. Discontinue on the second day of menstruation. It can be used this way on a monthly basis. For temporary relief from discomfort and irritability, enjoy a cup of ginkgo tea.

ABOUT PMS

❊ Studies have shown that women who regularly consume three or more cups of coffee daily are four times more likely than non or moderate coffee drinkers to have severe PMS.

❊ A significant number of PMS sufferers also have some type of thyroid dysfunction.

❊ Recent research suggests that some women who suffer from PMS may be deficient in melatonin. A hormone that regulates the body's biological clock, melatonin is secreted at night by the pineal gland.

❊ In Japan, women suffering from the effects of PMS drink kombuchu tea. This energizing beverage is high in antioxidants and immune-boosting phytochemicals.

❊ Many gynecologists recommend oral contraceptives for women with PMS. Oral contraceptives lessen PMS symptoms by "tricking" the body into believing it is pregnant.

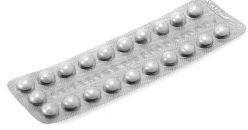

GROW IT YOURSELF

Ginkgo may have its roots in prehistoric China, but that hasn't stopped it from becoming a favorite of modern home gardeners and big city planners. An amazingly hardy tree, it displays attractive fan-shaped, medium green foliage and plumlike fruit. If you'd like to try growing this eye-catching tree yourself, be aware that it is slow-growing, often taking up to 20 years to reach 20 to 30 feet. However, when something is as gorgeous and as easy to care for as ginkgo, who cares if it takes its time growing up?

GINKGO BILOBA

Leaves improve the circulation.

• **Size.** Up to 120 feet high.

• **Native Habitat.** Dry, sunny to partially shady areas of China. It has been introduced to Australia, Europe, Korea, Japan, India and the United States, where it often thrives in urban parks and city sidewalk planters.

• **Cultivation.** Well adapted to poor, dry soil and polluted environments. Young ginkgo trees can be purchased from nurseries in sizes from 2 to 5 feet. Choose a preferably sunny, or partially sunny, area of your garden and plant tree in mid- to late spring after the last frost. Water sparingly and do not prune or fertilize plant for the first year. The tree should grow 6 to 12 inches the first year. A limited amount of leaves can be harvested at the end of the second summer. Note: If using your ginkgo leaves for medicinal purposes, do not treat the tree with pesticides.

GATHERING YOUR OWN

Hunting wild herbs is a satisfying introduction to herbal therapy—but when done thoughtlessly, it can cause plant extinction. In fact, today's increased interest in wild herb gathering has left many indigenous plants extinct; echinacea, ginger, ginseng, goldenseal, sweet grass, and wild carrot are now nearly impossible to find in their native habitats. Fortunately, ginkgo trees are abundant in many American cities—but to keep it that way, please ask yourself the following questions before gathering:

✔ Is this plant endangered? If so, it may be illegal in your state to gather it.

✔ Do I need to take this herb from the wild or can I purchase it or grow it myself?

✔ Am I gathering for personal use only and not for commercial use?
Note: Gathering wild plants for commercial use is illegal in many states.

✔ What part of the plant do I need? In the United States and Europe, the ginkgo's leaves are considered the medicinal portion of the ginkgo tree. Leaves are best gathered in late summer when their active compounds are at their most concentrated.

✔ What will I be using this herb for and exactly how much of it do I need?

✔ Is the ground wet where the tree is growing? If so, find trees growing in a dry spot or return when the ground is dry. Walking on wet soil compresses the dirt, making it difficult for future growth.

✔ Are the trees growing in sprayed areas, such as a city park sprayed with pesticides or marshes sprayed for mosquito control?

✔ Can I leave behind enough healthy leaves for the local animal population?

DO-IT-YOURSELF REMEDIES

❊ **Capsule:** Make your own herb supplements by purchasing animal or vegetable gelatin capsules at your local health food store and packing each individual capsule with 40 mg dried, powdered ginkgo leaves. **Standard dosage:** 1 capsule three times daily.

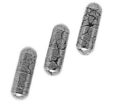

❊ **Drying:** Wash, thoroughly dry and chop fresh ginkgo leaves into small pieces. Lay the chopped herb on trays in a dry, well-ventilated, nonsunny area of your home or place in an extremely low oven, making sure air is continually circulating around the herbs. Or you can use a dehydrator. Drying will take between seven and 14 days. When drying herbs either in a warm room or an oven, the temperature should be kept between 70° to 90° F. Store dried root in a dark, airtight, nonporous container.

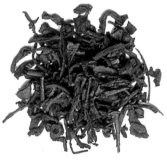

❊ **Fomentation:** Fomentations are essentially gauze or surgical bandages that are soaked in freshly made herbal tea. The hot cloth is then laid directly on a bite, rash or wound.

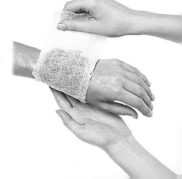

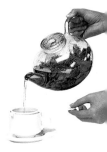

❊ **Infused Oil Made With Fresh Leaves:** Infused oils boast the fat-soluble active principles of whatever medicinal plant or herb was used to make them. One way to create ginkgo oil is to tightly pack a clean jar to its top with fresh ginkgo leaves. Pour almond or olive oil into the jar to cover the herb. Seal the jar tightly and leave in a warm place for six to seven weeks. Shake it daily. When ready to use, strain the oil and store in a dark, airtight container for up to two years. Can be ingested or used externally.

❊ **Liquid Extract.** Also known as extract. To make ginkgo extract, macerate 100 to 200 g of dried ginkgo leaves, or 300 to 500 g of fresh leaves. Place the herb in a jar and pour in 335 ml vodka (37 proof or higher) and 165 ml water. Place the lid on the jar and store in a dark area for four to eight weeks. Shake the mixture daily. When ready, strain the mixture, pressing all remaining liquid from the ginkgo leaves. Place liquid in a nonreactive saucepan and simmer over medium heat for 20 to 40 minutes until the liquid has been reduced by a third. This process burns off the alcohol, leaving the medicinal liquid behind. Allow liquid to cool and decant into several dropper bottles or a clean glass bottle. Will keep up to two years. Shake before using. **Standard dosage:** 5 ml three times a day.

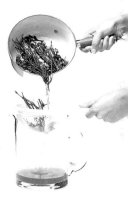

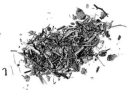

DO-IT-YOURSELF REMEDIES

❉ **Ointment:** Also called a salve, herbal ointment is easy to make at home. To create your own ginkgo ointment, mix 1 to 2 parts beeswax or soft paraffin wax, 7 parts cocoa butter, and 3 parts dried, powdered ginkgo leaves, in a nonreactive saucepan. Cook the mixture for one to two hours on a low setting. Let cool, package in an airtight container and apply up to three times a day.

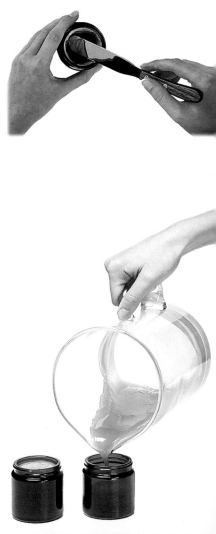

❉ **Poultice:** Fresh herbs can be applied directly to the skin when fashioned into a poultice. To make a ginkgo poultice, chop fresh or dried flowers and/or leaves. Boil in a small amount of water for 5 minutes (or use a microwave). Squeeze out any excess liquid from the boiled herb (reserve liquid). Lay the ginkgo leaves directly on the skin and cover with a warm moist towel. Leave in place for up to 30 minutes. The reserved liquid can be rewarmed and used to reheat the towel.

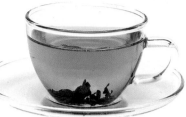

❋ **Tea:** Also known as an infusion, tea is an easy and common way to ingest an herb. To make ginkgo tea, steep 1 teaspoon dried ginkgo leaves or 1 tablespoon fresh leaves for five minutes in 1 cup of boiling water. You may add fructose, sugar, or honey to sweeten. **Standard dosage:** 1 cup of tea three times daily.

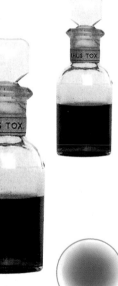

❋ **Tinctures:** Though they are not as potent as liquid extracts, tinctures are minimally processed, making them a favorite remedy among many herbalists. To make your own ginkgo tincture, place 100 to 200 grams of dried ginkgo leaves, or 300 to 500 grams of fresh ginkgo leaves, in a large jar and cover with 500 ml vodka (37 proof or higher). Place the lid on the jar and store in a dark area for four to six weeks. Shake the bottle daily. When ready to use, strain the mixture, pressing all remaining liquid from the leaves. Decant into several dropper bottles or a clean glass bottle. Will keep for up to a year.

ALTERNATIVE HEALTH STRATEGIES

Herbs, vitamins, minerals—sure these contribute to good health. But creating general well-being involves more than simply taking supplements. Good health has to do with various quality of life issues that can aggravate or cause stress, thus harming health. Here are some additional ways to help keep yourself well.

Improve Your Eating Habits

Here are the five main eating strategies people follow; consider finding the healthiest one that works with your lifestyle.

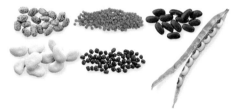

- **OMNIVORE**
- **PISCATORIAL**
- **MACROBIOTIC**
- **VEGAN**
- **VEGETARIAN**

Get More Exercise

Whether it's walking or weightlifting, any type of exercise can help you feel better. Try any of these types:

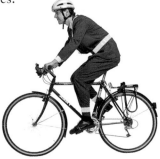

- **STRETCHING**
- **AEROBICS**
- **STRENGTH TRAINING**

Simple Ways To Ease Stress
In addition to exercise and healthy eating, here are some more
techniques–old and new–for easing stress and increasing relaxation.

- GET ENOUGH SLEEP
- MEDITATE REGULARLY
- GIVE UP JUNK FOOD
- ADOPT A PET
- SURROUND YOURSELF WITH SUPPORTIVE PEOPLE
- LIMIT YOUR EXPOSURE TO CHEMICALS
- TAKE YOUR VITAMINS
- ENJOY YOURSELF

ONE-MINUTE STRESS REDUCER
Stress is one of the top health hazards we face today.
Unfortunately, it's impossible to go through life without the
irritations that make us tense. Fortunately, there *is* something
you can do to minimize their power to aggravate you. It's
called deep breathing, and it can be done anywhere and
anytime you need to calm and center yourself. Here's how it
works:

1. Inhale deeply through your nose.
2. Hold your breath for up to three seconds, then
   exhale your breath through your mouth.
3. Continue as needed.

Deep breathing pulls a person's attention away from a given
stressor and refocuses it on his or her breath. This type of
breathing is not only comforting (thanks to its rhythmic
quality), but also has been shown to lower rapid pulse and
shallow respiration—two temporary symptoms of stress.

HERB GLOSSARY

After being used for centuries in Africa, Asia and Europe, herbs are finally making their way into American homes. Which is exactly where they belong. Herbs are good medicine. So good that many of our modern drugs are based on herbs' active ingredients. For example, the active component in aspirin is salicin, a biologically active ingredient of white willow bark. Salicin is also found in lesser amounts in birch bark and peppermint.

Herbal remedies come in a variety of forms, including dried and fresh leaves, capsules, liquid extracts, oils, teas, tinctures and more. Doses generally depend on the remedy's form and its potency. Currently there is no US government agency that checks the concentration of an herbal remedy's active ingredient. One of the best ways to ensure that you're getting what you pay for is to look for a product with a standardized extract. This guarantees that the remedy will contain the stated percentage of the herb's active ingredient.

One last note: Herbal remedies have an ancient track record for safety. However, they can cause harm when used incorrectly or by individuals with contraindications. If you are unsure of whether an herb is for you, please contact your physician or a naturopathic doctor.

ALOE

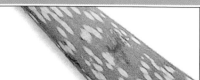

Properties: Analgesic, antibacterial, antifungal, anti-inflammatory, anti-itch, antiseptic, circulatory stimulant, digestive aid, immune-system stimulant, laxative.

Target Ailments: Acne, bruises, burns, constipation, cuts, insect bites, digestive disorders, rashes, ulcers, wounds.

Available Forms: Capsule, fresh leaves, gel, juice, liquid extract.

Possible Side Effects: When taken internally, aloe can cause severe cramping in some individuals.

Precautions: Pregnant women should not ingest aloe; It can stimulate uterine contractions.

CALENDULA

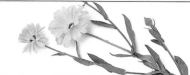

Properties: Antibacterial, anti-inflammatory, antiseptic, antispasmodic, promotes sweating, sedative.

Target Ailments: Burns, cuts, fungal infections, gallbladder conditions, hepatitis, indigestion, irregular menstruation, insect bites, menstrual cramps, mouth sores, skin rashes, ulcers, wounds.

Available Forms: Capsule, dried herb, fresh herb, liquid extract, lotion, oil, ointment, tincture.

Possible Side Effects: None expected.

Precautions: Calendula is related to ragweed. Individuals allergic to ragweed should consult a physician before using calendula.

ASTRAGALUS

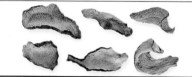

Properties: Antibacterial, anti-inflammatory, antioxidant, antiviral, diuretic, immune-system stimulant.

Target Ailments: Cancer, colds, appetite loss, diarrhea, fatigue, flu, heart conditions, HIV, viral infections.

Available Forms: Capsule, dried herb, fresh herb, liquid extract, tea, tincture.

Possible Side Effects: None expected.

Precautions: Astragalus should be used as a companion therapy to—not a replacement for—traditional cancer and HIV therapies.

CHAMOMILE

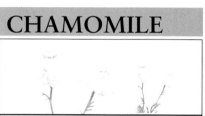

Properties: Antibacterial, anti-inflammatory, antiseptic, antispasmodic, carminative, digestive aid, fever reducer, sedative.

Target Ailments: Gingivitis, hemorrhoids, insomnia, indigestion, intestinal gas, menstrual cramps, nausea, nervousness, stomachaches, sunburns, tension, ulcers, varicose veins.

Available Forms: Capsule, dried herb, fresh herb, liquid extract, lotion, oil, tea, tincture.

Possible Side Effects: None expected.

Precautions: Because chamomile is related to ragweed, individuals with ragweed allergies should consult a physician before using chamomile.

DONG QUAI

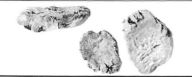

Properties: Antiallergenic, antispasmodic, diuretic, mild laxative, muscle relaxant, vasodilator.
Target Ailments: Abscesses, blurred vision, heart palpitations, irregular menstruation, light-headedness, menstrual pain, pallor, poor circulation.
Available Forms: Capsule, dried herb, liquid extract, tincture.
Possible Side Effects: Can cause photosensitivity in some individuals.
Precautions: Dong quai has abortive abilities; Do not take while pregnant.

FEVERFEW

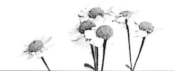

Properties: Anti-inflammatory, fever reducer.
Target Ailments: Arthritis, asthma, dermatitis, menstrual pain, migraines.
Available Forms: Capsule, dried herb, fresh herb, liquid extract, tincture.
Possible Side Effects: Some individuals experience "withdrawal" symptoms after taking feverfew, including fatigue and nervousness.
Precautions: Because it is related to ragweed, individuals with ragweed allergies should consult a physician before using feverfew.

ECHINACEA

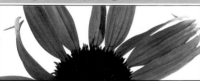

Properties: Antiallergenic, antibacterial, antiseptic, antimicrobial, antiviral, carminative, lymphatic tonic.
Target Ailments: Abscesses, acne, bladder infections, blood poisoning, burns, colds, eczema, food poisoning, flu, insect bites, kidney infections, mononucleosis, respiratory infections, sore throats.
Available Forms: Capsule, dried herb, liquid extract, tea, tincture.
Possible Side Effects: High doses can cause dizziness and nausea.
Precautions: Do not take echinacea for more than four weeks in a row.

GARLIC

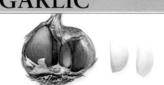

Properties: Antibacterial, anticoagulant, antifungal, anti-inflammatory, antiviral, cholesterol reducer, digestive aid, immune-system stimulant, worm-fighting.
Target Ailments: Arteriosclerosis, arthritis, bladder infections, colds, digestive upset, flu, heart conditions, high blood pressure, high blood cholesterol, viral infections.
Available Forms: Capsule, fresh cloves, liquid extract, oil, tincture.
Possible Side Effects: Can cause upset stomach.
Precautions: While garlic is safe taken in culinary doses, individuals on anticoagulant medications should consult their doctors before supplementing their diet with garlic.

GINGER

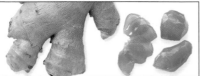

Properties: Antibacterial, anticoagulant, antinausea, antispasmodic, antiviral, carminative, digestive aid, expectorant, immune-system stimulant, muscle relaxant.
Target Ailments: Burns, colds, flu, high blood pressure, high cholesterol, liver conditions, intestinal gas, menstrual cramps, motion sickness, nausea, stomachaches.
Available Forms: Capsule, dried root, tea.
Possible Side Effects: Heartburn.
Precautions: While ginger is safe in culinary doses, individuals who suffer from a blood-clotting disorder or are on anticoagulant medication should consult a physician before supplementing their diet with the herb.

GINSENG

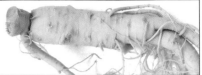

Properties: Antibacterial, antidepressant, immune-system stimulant, stimulant.
Target Ailments: Colds, depression, fatigue, flu, impaired immune system, respiratory conditions, stress.
Available Forms: Capsule, dried root, fresh root, liquid extract, tincture, tea.
Possible Side Effects: Large doses of ginseng can cause breast soreness, headaches or skin rashes in some individuals.
Precautions: Ginseng can aggravate existing heart palpitations or high blood pressure.

GINKGO BILOBA

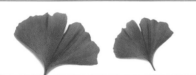

Properties: Antibacterial, anti-inflammatory, antioxidant, circulatory stimulant, vasodilator.
Target Ailments: Clotting disorders, dementia, depression, headaches, hearing loss, Raynaud's syndrome, tinnitus, vascular diseases, vertigo.
Available Forms: Capsule, dry herb, liquid extract, tincture, tea.
Possible Side Effects: Diarrhea, irritability, nausea, restlessness.
Precautions: Do not use ginkgo biloba if you have a blood-clotting disorder like hemophilia or are taking anticoagulant medications.

GOLDENSEAL

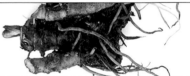

Properties: Antacid, antibacterial, antifungal, anti-inflammatory, antiseptic, astringent, digestive aid, stimulant.
Target Ailments: Canker sores, contact dermatitis, diarrhea, eczema, food poisoning.
Available Forms: Capsule, dry herb, liquid extract, tea, tincture.
Possible Side Effects: In high doses, goldenseal can cause diarrhea and nausea and can irritate the skin, mouth and throat.
Precautions: Because of its high cost, many manufacturers adulterate preparations with less costly herbs, such as barberry, yellow dock or bloodroot, some of which can cause unwanted reactions when taken in high doses.

KAVA

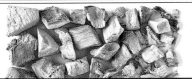

Properties: Antidepressant, antispasmodic, aphrodisiac, diuretic, muscle relaxant, sedative.

Target Ailments: Anxiety, colds, depression, menstrual conditions, muscle cramps, respiratory tract conditions, stress.

Available Forms: Capsule, dried herb, liquid extract, tea, tincture.

Possible Side Effects: Allergic skin reactions, muscle weakness, red eyes, sleepiness.

Precautions: In high doses, kava can impair motor reflexes and cause breathing problems.

MILK THISTLE

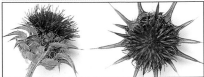

Properties: Anti-inflammatory, antioxidant, digestive aid, immune-system stimulant.

Target Ailments: inflammation of the gallbladder duct, hepatitis, liver conditions, poisoning from ingestion of the death cup mushroom, psoriasis.

Available Forms: Capsule, dried herb, fresh herb, powder, tea, tincture.

Possible Side Effects: Milk thistle can cause mild diarrhea when taken in large doses.

Precautions: If you think you have a liver disorder, seek medical advice before taking this herb.

LAVENDER

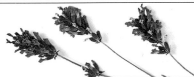

Properties: Antibacterial, antidepressant, antiseptic, antispasmodic, carminative, circulatory stimulant, digestive aid, diuretic, sedative.

Target Ailments: Anxiety, depression, headache, insomnia, intestinal gas, nausea, tension.

Available Forms: Capsule, dried herb, fresh herb, oil, tincture.

Possible Side Effects: Lavender products can cause skin irritation in sensitive individuals.

Precautions: Lavender oil is poisonous when ingested internally.

PARSLEY

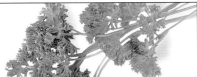

Properties: Antiseptic, antispasmodic, digestive aid, diuretic, laxative, muscle relaxant.

Target Ailments: Colds, congestion, fever, flu, indigestion, irregular menstruation, premenstrual syndrome, stimulating the production of breast milk, stomachaches.

Available Forms: Capsule, dried herb, fresh herb, liquid extract, oil, tea, tincture.

Possible Side Effects: Can cause photosensitivity in some individuals.

Precautions: Parsley should not be ingested in large amounts or used externally during pregnancy; it contains compounds that may stimulate uterine muscles and possibly cause miscarriage.

PEPPERMINT

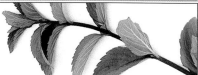

Properties: Antacid, antibacterial, antidepressant, antispasmodic, carminatve, expectorant, muscle relaxant, promotes sweating.
Target Ailments: Anxiety, colds, fever, flu, insomnia, intestinal gas, itching, migraines, morning sickness, motion sickness, nausea.
Available Forms: Capsule, dried herb, fresh herb, lozenge, oil, ointment, tea, tincture.
Possible Side Effects: When applied externally, peppermint products can cause skin reactions in sensitive individuals.
Precautions: If you have a hiatal hernia, talk to your doctor before using peppermint products externally or internally; the oil in the plant can exacerbate symptoms.

SAGE

Properties: Antiseptic, anti-inflammatory, antioxidant, antispasmodic, astringent, bile stimulant, carminative, reduces perspiration.
Target Ailments: Excess intestinal gas, insect bites, menopausal night sweats, poor circulation, reduces milk flow at weaning, sore throat, stomachaches, mouth ulcers.
Available Forms: Capsule, dried herb, fresh herb, liquid extract, oil, tincture.
Possible Side Effects: Sage tea may cause inflammation of the lips and/or tongue in some individuals.
Precautions: Do not ingest pure sage oil; it is toxic when taken internally.

ROSEMARY

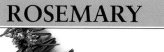
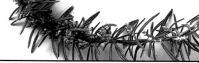

Properties: Antibacterial, antidepressant, anti-inflammatory, antiseptic, carminative, circulctory stimulant.
Target Ailments: Bad breath, dandruff, depression, eczema, headaches, indigestion, joint inflammation, mouth and throat infections, muscle pain, psoriasis, rheumatoid arthritis.
Available Forms: Dried herb, fresh herb, ingestible rosemary-flavored oil, oil, ointment, tea, tincture.
Possible Side Effects: Rosemary oil can cause skin inflammation and/or dermatitis.
Precautions: Do not mistake regular rosemary oil for ingestible rosemary-flavored oil.

SAW PALMETTO

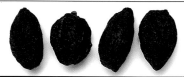

Properties: Antiallergenic, anti-inflammatory, diuretic, immune-boosting.
Target Ailments: Asthma, benign prostatic hyperplasia, bronchitis, colds, cystitis, impotence, male infertility, nasal congestion, sinus conditions, sore throats.
Available Forms: Capsule, dried herb, fresh herb, liquid extract, oil, tea, tincture.
Possible Side Effects: Can cause diarrhea if taken in large doses.
Precautions: Due to its hormonal actions, saw palmetto may interact negatively with prostate medicines or hormonal treatments such as estrogen replacement therapy, possibly canceling out their effectiveness.

ST. JOHN'S WORT

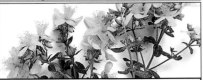

Properties: Analgesic, antibacterial, anti-depressant, anti-inflammatory, antiviral, astringent.
Target Ailments: Attention deficit disorder, anxiety, bacterial infections, burns, carpal tunnel syndrome, depression, HIV, menopause.
Available Forms: Capsule, dried herb, liquid extract, oil, ointment, tea, tincture.
Possible Side Effects: Gastrointestinal upset, headaches, photosensitivity, stiff neck.
Precautions: Avoid foods containing the amino acid tyramine when taking St. John's wort; the interaction of the two can cause an increase in blood pressure. Foods with tyramine include beer, coffee, wine, chocolate and fava beans.

WILD YAM

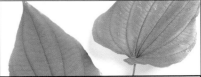

Properties: Analgesic, anti-inflammatory, antispasmodic, expectorant, muscle relaxant, promotes sweating.
Target Ailments: Menopause, menstrual cramps, morning sickness, nausea, rheumatoid arthritis, urinary tract infections.
Available Forms: Capsule, cream, dried root, liquid extract, oil, powder, tincture.
Possible Side Effects: Can cause vomiting in large doses.
Precautions: Individuals who are suffering from a hormone-sensitive cancer, such as breast or uterine cancer, should avoid wild yam. Some experts believe that the herb can encourage the growth of cancer cells.

VALERIAN

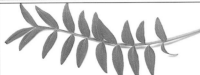

Properties: Analgesic, antibacterial, antispasmodic, carminative, reduces blood pressure, sedative, tranquilizer.
Target Ailments: Brachial spasm, high blood pressure, insomnia, palpitations, menstrual pain, migraines, muscle cramps, nervousness, tension headaches, wounds.
Available Forms: Capsules, dried herb, liquid extract, oil, teas, tincture.
Possible Side Effects: Headaches with prolonged use.
Precautions: Do not take with other sedatives, including alcohol. Do not drive or operate machinery after taking valerian.

YARROW

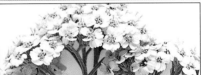

Properties: Antibacterial, anti-inflammatory, antispasmodic, blood coagulator, bile stimulating, immune-system stimulant, promotes sweating, sedative.
Target Ailments: Anxiety, colds and flu, cystitis, digestive disorders, menstrual cramps, minor wounds, nosebleeds, poor circulation, skin rashes.
Available Forms: Dried herb, capsule, liquid extract, oil, tea, tincture.
Possible Side Effects: Diarrhea, skin rash.
Precautions: Yarrow is related to ragweed and can cause an allergic reaction in individuals with ragweed allergies. Do not take if pregnant; it can induce miscarriage.

HERBAL TERMS

You're thumbing through the latest herbal therapy book when you run smack into the word "emmenagogue." Or perhaps you get tangled on "oxytocic." For anyone who's ever been stopped by an unfamiliar alternative medical term, we offer the following list:

Adaptogenic: Increases resistance and resilience to stress. Supports adrenal gland functioning.

Alterative: Blood purifier that improves the condition of the blood, improves digestion, and increases the appetite. Used to treat conditions arising from or causing toxicity.

Analgesic: Herb that relieves pain either by relaxing muscles or reducing pain signals to the brain.

Anthelmintic: Destroys or expels intestinal worms.

Antacid: Neutralizes excess stomach and intestinal acids.

Antiallergenic: Inactivates allergenic substances in the body.

Antibacterial/Antibiotic: Helps the body fight off harmful bacteria.

Antidepressant: Helps maintain emotional stability.

Anticatarrhal: Eliminates or counteracts the formation of mucus.

Anticoagulant: Thins blood and helps prevent blood clots.

Antifungal: Kills infection-causing fungi.

Anti-inflammatory: Reduces swelling of the tissues.

Anti-itch: Deadens itching sensations.

Antimicrobial: Kills a wide range of harmful bacteria, fungi, and viruses.

Antioxidant: Fights harmful oxidation.

Antipyretic/Fever Reducer: Reduces or prevents fever.

Antiseptic: External application prevents bacterial growth on skin.

Antispasmodic: Prevents or relaxes muscle tension.

Antiviral: Helps the body fight invading viruses.

Astringent: Has a constricting or binding effect. Commonly used to treat hemorrhages, secretions and diarrhea.

Blood Coagulant: Thickens blood and aids in clotting.

Carminative: Relieves gas.

Cholagogue: Encourages the flow of bile into the small intestine.

Circulatory Stimulant: Promotes even and efficient blood circulation.

Demulcent: Soothing substance, usually mucilage, taken internally to protect injured or inflamed tissues.

Diaphoretic: Induces sweating.

Diuretic: Increases urine flow.

Emetic: Induces vomiting.

Emmenagogue: Promotes menstruation.

Emollient: Softens, soothes and protects skin.

Expectorant: Assists in expelling mucus from the lungs and throat.

Galactogogue: Increases the secretion of breast milk.

Hemostatic: Stops hemorrhaging and encourages blood coagulation.

Hepatic: Tones and strengthens the liver.

Hypotensive: Lowers abnormally elevated blood pressure.

Immune-System Stimulant: Strengthens immune system so the body can fight off invading organisms.

Laxative: Promotes bowel movements.

Lithotriptic: Helps dissolve urinary and biliary stones.

Muscle Relaxant: Loosens tight muscles and reduces muscle cramping.

Nervine: Calms tension.

Oxytocic: Stimulates uterine contractions.

Rubefacient: Increases blood flow at the surface of the skin.

Sedative: Quiets the nervous system.

Sialagogue/Digestive Aid: Promotes the flow of saliva.

Stimulant: Increases the body's energy.

Tonic: Promotes the functions of body systems.

Vasoconstrictor: Constricts blood vessels, limiting the amount of blood flowing to a particular area.

Vasodilator: Dilates blood vessels, helping to promote blood flow.

Vulnerary: Encourages wound healing by promoting cell growth and repair.

HERBAL ORGANIZATIONS

Where to go for more information:

American Botanical Council
P.O. Box 201660
Austin, TX 78720
512-331-8868
www.herbalgram.org

The American Herbalist Guild
P.O. Box 746555
Arvada, CO 80006
303-423-8800

American Herbalists Guild
Box 1683
Soquel, CA 95073
408-464-2441

Herb Research Foundation
1007 Pearl Street, Suite 200
Boulder, CO 80302
303-449-2265
www.herbs.org

National Accupuncture and Oriental Medicine Alliance
14637 Starr Road SE
Olalla, WA 98359
206-851-6896

National Institutes of Health Office of Alternative Medicine
9000 Rockville Pike
Building 31, Room 5B-37
Mailstop 2182
Bethesda, MD 20892
301-402-2466

The Herb Society of America
9019 Kirtland-Chardon Road
Kirtland, OH 44094
216-256-0514

American College of Sports Medicine
P.O. Box 1440
Indianapolis, IN 46206
317-637-9200

American Heart Association
7272 Greenville Avenue
Dallas, TX 75231
214-373-6300

National Health Information Center
P.O. Box 1133
Washington, DC 20013
800-336-4797

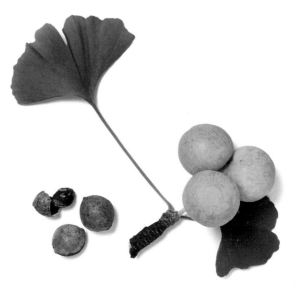

GROWING HERBS

Interested in cultivating herbs yourself?
These sources can supply roots, plants, and/or seeds.

Catoctin Mountain Botanicals
P.O. Box 454
Jefferson, MD 21755
301-473-4351

Companion Plants
7247 N. Coolville Ridge Rd.
Athens, OH 45701
614-593-3092
E-mail: complants@frognet.net

Dry Fork Herb Gardens
R.R.#1 Box 21
Rockport, IL
217-437-5281

Ecofriendly Farms
15488 Barn Rock Rd.
Mendota, VA 24270
540-466-8689

Goodwin Creek Gardens
P.O. Box 83
Williams, OR 97544
541-846-7357

Herbal Exchange
P.O. Box 429
9160 Lentz Rd.
Frazeysburg, OH 43822
614-828-9968

Horizon Herbs
P.O. Box 69
Williams, OR 97544
541-846-6233
www.chatlink.com/~herbseed
E-mail: herbseed@chatlink.com

Johnny's Seeds
Rt. 1 Box 2580
Foss Hill Rd.
Albion, ME 04910
207-437-9294
www.johnnyseeds.com

Mountain Traditions
H.C. 68, Box 193
Big Creek, KY 40914
606-598-6904

Nature's Cathedral
Rt. 1 Box 120
Blairstown, IA 52209
319-454-6959

Prairie Moon Nursery
Rt. 3, Box 163
Winona, MN 55987
507-452-1362

Wilcox Natural Products
P.O. Box 391
755 George Wilson Rd.
Boone, NC 28607
828-264-3615
www.goldenseal.com

Wild Wonderful Farm, Inc.
P.O. Box 256
Franklin, WV 26268
212-736-1467

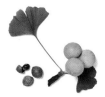

INDEX

ABOUT THE AUTHOR

Stephanie Pedersen is a writer and editor who specializes in the area of health. Her articles have appeared in numerous publications, including *American Woman, Sassy, Teen, Weight Watchers* and *Woman's World*. She has also co-written *What Your Cat is Trying to Tell You: A Head-to-Tail Guide to Your Cat's Symptoms and Their Solutions* and *What Your Dog is Trying to Tell You: A Head-to-Tail Guide to Your Dog's Symptoms and Their Solutions,* both published by St. Martin's Press. She currently resides in New York City.

Picture Credits: Steve Gorton, David Murray, Dave King, Martin Norris, Philip Gatward, Andy Crawford, Philip Dowell, Clive Streeter, Peter Chadwick, Tim Ridley, Andrew Whittack, Martin Cameron

DORLING KINDERSLEY PUBLISHING, INC.
www.dk.com

Published in the United States by
Dorling Kindersley Publishing, Inc.
95 Madison Avenue • New York, New York 10016

Editorial Director: LaVonne Carlson
Editors: Nancy Burke, Barbara Minton, Connie Robinson
Designer: Carol Wells
Cover Designer: Gus Yoo

Pedersen, Stephanie.
    Ginkgo biloba : ease anxiety and increase intellect / by Stephanie
Pedersen. – 1st American ed.
    p.   cm. -- (Natural care library)
    Includes index.
    ISBN 0-7894-5188-3 (alk. paper)
    1. Ginkgo--Therapeutic use   I. Title. II. Series.
RM666.G489P43 2000
615'. 3257--dc21
99-41997